Menopau

Plan

Instructional manual on the causes, symptoms, treatments, prevention of premenopause (Natural hormone balance)

Barbara S. Johnson

Table of Contents

INTRODUCTION

Menopause is enough time that marks the finish of your menstrual cycles. It's diagnosed after you have gone a year with out a menstrual period. Menopause can occur in your 40s or 50s, however the average age group is 51 in america.

Menopause is an all natural biological process. However the physical symptoms, such as hot flashes, and psychological symptoms of menopause may disrupt your rest, decrease your energy or impact psychological health. There are numerous effective treatments available, from lifestyle modifications to hormone therapy.

Chapter 1

Menopause

Menopause is enough time that marks the finish of your menstrual cycles. It's diagnosed after you have gone a year with out a menstrual period. Menopause can occur in your 40s or 50s, however the average age group is 51 in america.

Menopause is an all natural biological process. However the physical symptoms, such as hot flashes, and psychological symptoms of menopause may disrupt your rest, decrease your energy or impact psychological health. There are numerous effective treatments available, from lifestyle modifications to hormone therapy.

Causes

Menopause can derive from:

- Natural decline of reproductive hormones. As you strategise your past due 30s, your ovaries start making less estrogen and progesterone - the bodily hormones that control menstruation - as well as your fertility declines. Within your 40s, your menstrual period may become much longer or shorter, heavier or lighter, and pretty much frequent, till - normally, by age group 51 - your ovaries stop producing eggs, and also you haven't any more period.

- Hysterectomy. A hysterectomy that gets rid of your uterus however, not your ovaries usually doesn't cause immediate menopause. Although so long as have period, your ovaries still release eggs and produce estrogen and progesterone. But surgery that gets rid of both your uterus as well as your ovaries (total hysterectomy and bilateral oophorectomy) will cause immediate menopause. Your period stop immediately, and you might have hot flashes and other menopausal signs or symptoms, which may be severe, as these hormone changes happen abruptly rather than over many years.

- Chemotherapy and rays therapy. These malignancy therapies can induce menopause, leading to symptoms such as hot flashes during or soon after the treatment. The halt to menstruation (and fertility) is not necessarily permanent pursuing chemotherapy, so contraceptive measures may be desired.

- Main ovarian insufficiency. About 1 percent of women experience menopause before age group 40 (early menopause). Menopause may derive from main ovarian insufficiency - whenever your ovaries neglect to produce normal degrees of reproductive human hormones - stemming from hereditary factors or autoimmune disease. But often no cause are available. For these women, hormone therapy is normally suggested at least before natural age group of menopause to be able to protect the mind, heart and bone fragments.

When does menopause start and exactly how long will it last?

Nearly all women first start developing menopause symptoms about four years before their last period. Symptoms often continue until about four years after a woman's last period.

A small amount of women experience menopause symptoms for ten years before menopause actually occurs, and 1 in 10 women experience menopausal symptoms for 12 years following their last period.

The median age for menopause is 51, though it could occur typically up to 2 yrs earlier for African-American and Latina women. More studies are had a need to understand the onlist of menopause for non-Caucasian women.

There are several factors that help determine when you'll start menopause, including genetics and ovary health. Perimenopause occurs before menopause. Perimenopause is a period when your bodily hormones begin to improve in planning for menopause.

It could last from a couple of months to many years. A lot of women start perimenopause some point after their middle-40s. Other women miss perimenopause and enter menopause all of a sudden.

About 1 percent of women start menopause prior to the age of 40, to create premature menopause or primary ovarian insufficiency. About 5 percent of women go through menopause between your age groups of 40 and 45. That is known as early menopause.

Perimenopause vs. menopause versus. postmenopause

- During perimenopause, menstrual periods become irregular. Your period may be past due, or you might completely skip a number of periods. Menstrual circulation could also become heavier or lighter.

- Menopause is thought as too little menstruation for just one full year.

- Postmenopause identifies the years after menopause has occurred.

C h a p t e r   2

What exactly are the symptoms of menopause?

Every woman's menopause experience is exclusive. Symptoms are usually more serious when menopause occurs abruptly or higher a shorter time frame.

Conditions that impact the fitness of the ovary, like malignancy or hysterectomy, or certain lifestyle options, like smoking, have a tendency to increase the intensity and period of symptoms.

Apart from menstruation changes, the symptoms of perimenopause, menopause, and postmenopause are usually the same. The most frequent early indicators of perimenopause are:

- less regular menstruation.

- heavier or lighter period than you normally experience

- vasomotor symptoms, including hot flashes, night time sweats, and flushing

Around 75 percent of women experience hot flashes with menopause.

Other common symptoms of menopause include:

1. Insomnia.

2. Vaginal dryness.

3. Weight gain.

4. Depression.

5. Anxiety.

6. Difficulty concentrating.

7. Memory problems.

8. Reduced libido, or libido.

9. Dry skin, mouth area, and eyes.

10. Increased urination.

11. Sore or sensitive breasts.

12. Headaches.

13. Racing heart.

14. Urinary system infections (utis).

15. Reduced muscle tissue.

16. Unpleasant or stiff joints.

17. Reduced bone mass.

18. Less full breasts.

19. Loss hair or loss.

20. Increased hair regrowth on the areas of your body, like the face, neck, chest, and spine

Complications

Common problems of menopause include:

- Vulvovaginal atrophy.

- Dyspareunia, or painful intercourse.

- Slower metabolic function.

- Osteoporosis, or weaker bone fragments with minimal mass and strength.

- Mood or unexpected emotional changes.

- Cataracts.

- Periodontal disease.

- Urinary incontinence.

- Heart or bloodstream vessel disease

How come menopause occur?

Menopause is an all natural process occurring as the ovaries age group and produce less reproductive human hormones.

The body starts to endure several changes in response to lessen degrees of:

- Estrogen.

- Progesterone.

- Testosterone.

- Follicle-stimulating hormone (fsh).

- Luteinizing hormone (lh)

Probably one of the most well known changes is the increased loss of dynamic ovarian follicles. Ovarian follicles will be the constructions that produce and release eggs from the ovary wall structure, allowing menstruation and fertility.

The majority of females first spot the frequency of their period becoming less consistent, as the movement becomes heavier and longer. This usually occurs sooner or later in the mid-to-late 40s. By age 52, most U.S. women have undergone menopause.

In some instances, menopause is induced, or triggered by injury or surgery of the ovaries and related pelvic structures.

Common factors behind induced menopause include:

- bilateral oophorectomy, or surgery of the ovaries

- ovarian ablation, or the shutdown of ovary function, which might be done by hormone therapy, surgery, or radiotherapy techniques in women with estrogen receptor-positive tumors

- pelvic radiation

- pelvic injuries that severely damage or destroy the ovaries

How is menopause diagnosed?

It's worth speaking with your doctor if you're experiencing troublesome or disabling menopause symptoms, or you're experiencing menopause symptoms and are 45 years or younger.

A new bloodstream test known as the PicoAMH Elisa diagnostic test was recently approved by the meals and Drug AdministrationTrusted Source. This test is utilized to help determine whether a female has joined menopause or gets close to getting into menopause.

This new test may be beneficial to women who show

symptoms of perimenopause, which can likewise have adverse health impacts. Early menopause is associated with an increased threat of osteoporosis and fracture, cardiovascular disease, cognitive changes, genital changes and lack of libido, and feeling changes.

Your physician can also order a bloodstream test that will gauge the degree of certain bodily hormones in the bloodstream, usually FSH and a kind of estrogen called estradiol.

Regularly elevated FSH blood degrees of 30 mIU/mL or more, combined with too little menstruation for just one consecutive year, is usually confirmation of menopause. Saliva assessments and over-the-counter (OTC) urine assessments are also available, but they're unreliable and expensive.

During perimenopause, FSH and estrogen quantity fluctuate daily, so most health care providers will identify this condition predicated on symptoms, health background, and menstrual information.

Based on your symptoms and health background, your

doctor could also order additional blood vessels checks to help eliminate other root conditions which may be accountable for your symptoms.

Additional blood tests popular to help confirm menopause include:

- thyroid function tests

- bloodstream lipid profile

- liver function tests

- kidney function tests

- testosterone, progesterone, prolactin, estradiol, and chorionic gonadotropin (hCG) tests

Treatments

You might need treatment if your symptoms are severe or inside your standard of living. Hormone therapy may be a highly effective treatment in women under age 60, or within a decade of menopause onlist, for the decrease or management of:

- hot flashes

- night sweats

- flushing

- vaginal atrophy

- osteoporosis

Other medications enable you to treat more specific menopause symptoms, like hair loss and genital dryness.

Additional medications sometimes used for menopause medical indications include:

- topical minoxidil 5 percent, used once daily for baldness and loss

- antidandruff shampoos, commonly ketoconazole 2 percent and zinc pyrithione 1 percent, used for hair loss

- eflornithine hydrochloride topical cream for unwanted hair regrowth

- selective serotonin reuptake inhibitors (SSRIs),

commonly paroxetine 7.5 milligrams for hot flashes, anxiety, and depression

- non-hormonal genital moisturizers and lubricants

- low-dose estrogen-based genital lubricants by means of a cream, band, or tablet

- ospemifene for vaginal dryness and painful intercourse

- prophylactic antibiotics for repeated UTIs

- sleep medications for insomnia

- denosumab, teriparatide, raloxifene, or calcitonin for postmenstrual osteoporosis

Home cures and changes in lifestyle

There are many ways to lessen minor-to-moderate menopause symptoms normally, using home cures, changes in lifestyle, and alternative treatments.

Below are a few at-home methods for managing menopause symptoms:

Keeping cool and remaining comfortable

Clothe themselves in loose, layered clothing, especially through the nighttime and during warm or unpredictable weather. This assists you manage hot flashes.

Maintaining your bedroom cool and staying away from heavy blankets during the night can also lessen your likelihood of night sweats. In the event that you regularly have evening sweats, consider using a waterproof sheet under your bed linens to safeguard your mattress.

You can even carry a lightweight fan to help cool you down if you're feeling flushed.

Working out and managing your bodyweight

Lessen your daily calorie consumption by 400 to 600 calories to help control your bodyweight. It's also important to exercise reasonably for 20 to thirty minutes a day. This assists:

- increase energy

- promote a much better night's sleep

- improve mood

- promote your present well-being

Communicating your needs

Speak to a therapist or psychologist about any emotions of depression, stress, sadness, isolation, insomnia, and identification changes.

It's also advisable to try speaking with your loved ones members, family members, or friends about emotions of anxiety, mood changes, or depressive disorder in order that they know your preferences.

Vitamining your diet

Take calcium, vitamin D, and magnesium vitamins in reducing your risk for osteoporosis and improve energy and sleep. Speak to your doctor about vitamins that will help you for your own health needs.

Training relaxation techniques

Practice rest and deep breathing techniques, such as:

- yoga

- box breathing

- meditation

Caring for your skin

Apply moisturizers daily to lessen skin dryness. It's also advisable to avoid extreme bathing or going swimming, which can dry or irritate your skin layer.

Managing sleeping issues

Use OTC rest medications to temporarily manage your insomnia or consider discussing natural rest aids with your physician. Speak to your doctor if you regularly have sleep problems to allow them to help you manage it and get a much better night's rest.

Quitting smoking and restricting alcohol use

Stop smoking and prevent contact with secondhand smoke. Contact with cigarettes could make your symptoms even worse.

It's also advisable to limit your alcohol intake to lessen worsening symptoms. Heavy taking in during menopause may boost your risk of health issues.

Other remedies

Some limited studies have backed the utilization of herbal treatments for menopausal symptoms caused by estrogen deficiency.

Vitamins and nutrients that might help limit menopause medical indications include:

- soy

- vitamin E

- isoflavone

- melatonin

- flax seed

There's also claims that black cohosh may improve some symptoms, such as hot flashes and night sweats. However in a current overview of studies, little proof was found to aid these statements. More research is necessary.

Likewise, researchTrusted Source from 2015 found no evidence to aid claims that omega-3 essential fatty acids can improve vasomotor symptoms associated with menopause.

Outlook

Menopause is the natural cessation, or stopping, of the woman's menstrual period, and marks the finish of fertility. Majority of the women experience menopause by age 52, but pelvic or ovarian harm may cause unexpected menopause previously in life. Genetics or root conditions could also business lead to early starting point of menopause.

A lot of women experience menopause symptoms in the couple of years before menopause, mostly hot flashes, night sweats, and flushing. Symptoms can continue for four or even more years after menopause.

You may reap the benefits of treatment, such as hormone therapy, if your symptoms are severe or affect yourself. Generally, menopause symptoms can be handled or reduced using natural treatments and lifestyle changes.

Chapter 3

11 Natural Methods to Reduce Symptoms of Menopause

Menopause starts in the past due 40s or early 50s for some women. It usually continues for a couple of years.

During this time period, at least two-thirds of women experience the symptoms of menopause.

Included in these are hot flashes, night time sweats, disposition swings, irritability and fatigue.

Furthermore, menopausal women are in a higher threat of several diseases including osteoporosis, obesity, cardiovascular disease and diabetes.

Many women consider vitamins and remedies for relief.

This is a list of 11 natural ways to lessen the symptoms of menopause.

1. Eat Foods Abundant with Calcium and Vitamin D

Hormone changes during menopause can cause bone fragments to weaken, increasing the chance of osteoporosis.

Calcium and vitamin D are associated with good bone health, so it is important to get enough of the nutrients in what you eat.

Adequate vitamin D intake in postmenopausal women is also associated with a lesser threat of hip fractures credited to weak bone fragments.

Many foods are calcium-rich, including milk products like yogurt, milk and cheese.

Green, leafy vegetables such as kale, collard greens and spinach have lots of calcium mineral too. It is also abundant in tofu, coffee beans, sardines and other food stuffs.

Additionally, calcium-fortified foods are also good sources, including certain cereals, juice or milk alternatives.

Sunlight is your primary source of vitamin D, as your

epidermis produces it when subjected to sunlight. However, as you grow older, your skin layer gets less effective at rendering it.

In the event that you aren't out in sunlight much or if you hide your skin layer, either going for a product or increasing food resources of vitamin D may make a difference.

Rich nutritional sources include greasy fish, eggs, cod liver organ oil and foods fortified with vitamin D.

Important Thing:

A diet abundant with calcium mineral and vitamin D is important to avoid the bone reduction that may appear during menopause.

2. Achieve and keep maintaining a healthy weight

It's common to get weight during menopause.

This is due to a mixture of changing hormones, aging, lifestyle and genetics.

Gaining excess surplus fat, especially round the waist,

raises your threat of developing diseases such as cardiovascular disease and diabetes.

In addition, your weight may affect your menopause symptoms.

One research of 17,473 postmenopausal women discovered that those who lost at least 10 lbs (4.5 kg) of weight or 10% of their bodyweight over a 12 months were much more likely to remove hot flashes and evening sweats.

Here's more information about slimming down during menopause.

Important Thing:

Achieving and keeping a wholesome weight can help relieve menopause symptoms and assist in preventing disease.

3. Eat Plenty of Fruit and veggies

A diet abundant with fruits & vegetables can assist in preventing lots of menopause symptoms.

Fruits and vegetables are lower in calorie consumption and can help you are feeling full, so they're ideal for weight reduction and weight maintenance.

They could also assist in preventing lots of diseases, including cardiovascular disease.

That is important, since cardiovascular disease risk will increase after menopause. This may be credited to factors such as age group, putting on weight or perhaps reduced estrogen quantity.

Finally, vegetables & fruits also may help prevent bone loss.

One observational research of 3,236 women aged 50-59 discovered that diets saturated in fruit and veggies can lead to less bone break down.

Important Thing:

A diet abundant with fruit and veggies can help keep bone fragments healthy, and can assist in preventing putting on weight and certain diseases.

4. Avoid Result in Foods

Particular foods may trigger hot flashes, night time sweats and feeling swings.

They might be even much more likely to trigger you when you take in them during the night.

Common triggers include caffeine, alcohol and foods that are sweet or spicy.

Keep an indicator diary. In the event that you feel that one foods result in your menopause symptoms, make an effort to reduce your usage or prevent them completely.

Important Thing:

Particular foods and beverages can trigger hot flashes, evening sweats and disposition swings. This include caffeine, alcoholic beverages and sweet or spicy foods.

5. Exercise Regularly

There happens to be insufficient evidence to verify whether exercise works well for treating hot flashes and night sweats.

However, there is certainly evidence to aid other

advantages of regular exercise.

Included in these are improved energy and metabolism, healthier important joints and bone fragments, decreased stress and better rest.

For instance, one study discovered that working out three hours weekly for one 12 months improved physical and mental health insurance and overall standard of living in several menopausal women.

Regular physical exercise is also associated with better health insurance and protection against diseases and conditions including cancer, cardiovascular disease, stroke, high blood circulation pressure, type 2 diabetes, obesity and osteoporosis.

Important Thing:

Regular physical exercise can help alleviate menopause symptoms such as poor sleep, anxiety, low mood and fatigue. Additionally, it may protect against putting on weight and different diseases and conditions.

6. Eat Even More Foods That Are Saturated In

Phytoestrogens

Phytoestrogens are naturally occurring flower substances that can mimic the consequences of estrogen in the torso.

Therefore, they could help balance hormones.

The high intake of phytoestrogens in Parts of asia such as Japan is regarded as the key reason why menopausal ladies in these places hardly ever experience hot flashes.

Foods abundant with phytoestrogens include soybeans and soy products, tofu, tempeh, flaxseeds, linseeds, sesame seed products and coffee beans. However, the phytoestrogen content in foods varies depending on digesting methods.

One study discovered that diets saturated in soy were associated with minimal cholesterol quantity, blood circulation pressure and reduced severity of hot flashes and night time sweats among women who have been beginning to enter menopause.

However, the debate proceeds over whether soy products are good or harmful to you.

Evidence shows that real food resources of phytoestrogens are much better than vitamins or processed food items with added soy protein.

Important Thing:

Foods abundant with phytoestrogens may have modest benefits for hot flashes and cardiovascular disease risk. However, the data is mixed.

7. Drink Sufficient Water

During menopause, women often experience dryness. This really is likely triggered by the reduction in estrogen quantity.

Drinking 8-12 cups of water each day can help with these symptoms.

Normal water can also decrease the bloating that may appear with hormone changes.

Furthermore, water can assist in preventing putting on weight and assist in weight loss by assisting you feel full and increasing metabolism slightly.

Consuming 17 oz (500 ml) of drinking water, thirty minutes before meals may cause you to consume 13% fewer calories through the food.

Important Thing:

Drinking enough drinking water can help prevent putting on weight, assist in weight reduction and reduce symptoms of dryness.

8. Reduce Refined Sugars And Processed Food Items

A diet saturated in refined carbs and sugars can cause clear increases and dips in bloodstream glucose, causing you to feel tired and irritable.

Actually, one study discovered that diets saturated in processed carbs may boost the threat of depression in postmenopausal women.

Diets saturated in processed foods could also influence bone health.

A big observational study discovered that among women aged 50-59 years, diets saturated in processed and snacks were associated with poor bone quality.

Important Thing:

Diets saturated in processed food items and refined carbs are associated with an increased risk of major depression and even worse bone health in postmenopausal women.

9. Don't Miss Meals

Eating regular meals may make a difference when you're dealing with menopause.

Irregular eating could make certain symptoms of menopause even worse, and could even hinder weight loss efforts.

A year-long weight reduction program for postmenopausal women discovered that missing out meals was associated with 4.3% less weight reduction.

Important Thing:

Irregular eating could cause some symptoms of menopause to worsen. Missing out meals could also hinder weight reduction in postmenopausal women.

10. Eat Protein-Rich Foods

Regularly eating protein during the day can assist in preventing the increased loss of lean body mass occurring with age.

One study discovered that consuming protein each day at each meal may decelerate muscle loss due to aging.

Furthermore to helping prevent muscle loss, high-protein diets can help with weight loss because they promote fullness and raise the amount of calories burnt.

Foods abundant with protein include meats, seafood, eggs, legumes, nut products and dairy.

Important Thing:

Regular intake of high-quality protein may avoid the loss of muscle, assist in weight loss and help regulate mood and sleep.

11. Take VITAMINS

A lot of women take natural basic products and remedies to alleviate their menopause symptoms.

Unfortunately, the data behind most of them is weak.

Here are the most typical vitamins for reducing symptoms of menopause:

1. Phytoestrogens: These can be consumed through natural food resources or vitamins such as red clover components. There happens to be not enough proof to recommend them for alleviating menopause symptoms.

2. Black cohosh: Even though some studies discovered that dark cohosh may effectively alleviate hot flashes, the data is mixed. Furthermore, there's an insufficient long-term data on the security of this product.

3. Other vitamins: Proof is scarce for the potency of other widely used vitamins such as probiotics, prebiotics, kava, DHEA-S, dong quai and evening primrose oil.

Important Thing:

Natural vitamins can help treat menopause symptoms,

but more evidence is necessary about their safety and effectiveness

6 Foods In Order To Avoid During Menopause

Foods That May Worsen Menopausal Symptoms

1. Processed Foods

Poker chips and cookies might flavor good, but they're usually saturated in sodium, packed with added sugar, or both, which will make you retain drinking water and feel bloated, Jamieson-Petonic says. If you're craving a treat, get one of these healthier option, like string cheese, carrots dipped in hummus, or a few whole-grain crackers with peanut butter - they'll fulfill your need to nibble without filling up you up with the symptom-trigger stuff.

2. Spicy Foods

Think before you add that extra-hot salsa to your taco. Foods that rate on top of the heat level can cause sweating, flushing, and other symptoms of hot flashes, based on the Country wide Institute on Ageing. If you're seeking to then add kick to a bland dish, Jamieson-Petonic suggests missing the jalapeñoperating system and sprinkling on spices offering taste without as much warmth, like cumin, curry, turmeric, and basil.

3. Fast Food

In a rush? Drive-through restaurants may be convenient when you're brief promptly, but their foods often offer an enormous amount of excess fat, Jamieson-Petonic says. Fatty foods can boost your risk for cardiovascular disease, a condition that ladies already are at higher risk for after moving through menopause, based on the American Center Association. "These food types also have a tendency to promote putting on weight, which can exacerbate menopause symptoms as well," Jamieson-Petonic says. The better solution? Have quick, well balanced meals readily available by freezing leftovers at home or packaging a lunch. When you have to eat meals on the travel, miss the cheeseburger and choose healthier menu options. A grilled poultry sandwich on the whole-grain bun with lettuce and tomato is an excellent alternate, she says.

4. Alcohol

Although it might not be essential to swear off all cocktails and wine, there are many reasons to keep the alcohol consumption moderate. As recommended in the 2015-2020 U.S. Diet Guidelines for People in america, moderate drinking for ladies is thought as one drink each day or less. Women who've two to five beverages per day have 1.5 times the chance for breast cancer as those who don't drink whatsoever, and heavy consuming can boost your risk for coronary disease, based on the UNITED STATES Menopause Society. Plus, some women find that alcoholic beverages makes them more vunerable to hot flashes, Jamieson-Petonic says.

"I show women to hear their bodies," she says. "If alcoholic beverages aggravates their menopause symptoms they ought to stay away from it." In the event that you still want to indulge sometimes, Jamieson-Petonic suggests attempting a white wines spritzer with fruits, which is leaner in alcoholic beverages than most standard beverages.

5. Caffeine

Love your early morning glass of joe? Maybe it's worsening your menopause symptoms. A Mayo Medical center study released in Feb 2015 in the journal Menopause discovered that menopausal women who consumed caffeine were much more likely to have hot flashes than women who didn't consume caffeine. If you're craving a warm drink, get one of these glass of hot ginger or peppermint tea - both caffeine-free - Jamieson-Petonic says. Or if you're looking for a little extra energy, try taking a quick walk rather than counting on caffeine for a kick.

Fatty Meats

Besides being saturated in saturated body fat, foods like brisket and bacon can lower the body's serotonin quantity, Jamieson-Petonic says. "When serotonin drops, we feel uplist, grumpy, and irritable," she says. When you're searching for meats, miss the oily, marbled cuts and only trimmer alternatives, like poultry, turkey, and floor meat that's 90 percent slim or better.

The foodstuffs that are healthy during menopause are healthy at any stage in your daily life. Build healthy diet plan now and you'll enjoy better health for a long time to come, including through menopause.

Chapter 4

7 Best Foods for Menopause

Menopause is an all natural phase of each woman's life. However the side effect of fluctuating human hormones feel not normal. Additionally, hormone changes during menopause boost the threat of serious diseases, including osteoporosis, malignancy, and coronary disease. But upping your intake of the next seven foods can help.

1. Buckwheat

Buckwheat technically a seed (not really a wholegrain), buckwheat is a great source of organic carbs, needed for serotonin, a neurotransmitter associated with memory space and mood.

Theoretically a seed (not really a wholegrain), buckwheat is a great way to obtain complex carbs, needed for serotonin, a neurotransmitter associated with memory and mood. Studies also show that complicated carbs help reduce despression symptoms and elevate feeling.

Relating to other research, using a carb-containing food at supper may shorten rest starting point. Buckwheat is gluten-free and abundant with B nutritional vitamins, which also impact disposition.

Try out this: Stir-fry cooked buckwheat with eggs, green onions, carrots, ginger, and tamari for a twist on fried grain; toss prepared buckwheat with cut parsley, red onions, feta cheese, Kalamata olives, and essential olive oil; soak uncooked buckwheat, chia seed products, and coconut dairy overnight, then provide with berries and honey as an instant breakfast.

2. Collard greens

One glass of collards has as much calcium as a cup of milk, plus some studies suggest the absorption of calcium from vegetables is doubly high as from dairy.

Calcium is vital during menopause; osteoporosis impacts one of three postmenopausal women, as well as for those women, the life time threat of fractures is greater than the chance of breast malignancy. One glass of collards has as much calcium mineral as a glass of milk, plus some studies suggest the absorption of calcium mineral from vegetables is doubly high as from dairy products. Plus, collards are abundant with vitamin K and magnesium, also crucial for bone health.

Try out this: Sauté shredded collard greens, chickpeas, and garlic clove in essential olive oil and harissa; rip collard leaves into chip-sized items, toss with essential olive oil and sodium, and roast until crispy; therapeutic massage thinly sliced up collard leaves with essential olive oil and vinegar, then toss with radishes, lovely onions, and crumbled feta cheese for an instant salad.

3. Sardines

Like salmon, tuna, and other fatty seafood, sardines are saturated in omega-3 essential fatty acids, which can assist in preventing hot flashes and decrease the threat of osteoporosis and breasts cancer.

Like salmon, tuna, and other fatty seafood, sardines are saturated in omega-3 essential fatty acids, which can assist in preventing hot flashes and decrease the threat of osteoporosis and breasts cancer. Omega-3 fat also reduce triglyceride quantity and protect the heart-especially very important to women getting hormone therapy, which can increase triglyceride quantity. And if you take in canned sardines with bone fragments, you'll also be getting calcium mineral.

Try out this: Blend canned sardines with breads crumbs, minced onions, chopped parsley, and eggs, form into patties, and make in essential olive oil; in a food processor chip, combine smoked sardines, yogurt, smoked paprika, and dark pepper, process until just easy, and serve with vegetables for dipping; pass on mashed avocado on toast, coating with grilled onions and sardines, and sprinkle with parsley.

4. Flaxseeds

Flaxseeds will be the richest way to obtain lignans-phytoestrogens that are structurally much like estrogens and could reduce breast malignancy risk.

Flaxseeds will be the richest way to obtain lignans-phytoestrogens that are structurally just like estrogens and could reduce breast malignancy risk. Flax in addition has been shown to lessen evening sweats and hot flashes and improve standard of living during menopause. In a few studies, 40 grms each day of flaxseed experienced effects comparable to hormone alternative therapy for reducing menopausal symptoms.

Try out this: Defeat surface flaxseeds with buckwheat flour, honey, and eggs, and make silver-dollar pancakes; mix floor flax with sunflower seed products, basil, garlic clove, arugula, and lemon for a nut-free pesto; blend flaxseeds with chia seed products, coconut dairy, and coconut sugars, then top with raw cacao nibs and toasted coconut potato chips.

5. Tomato Sauce

Tomato sauce is a concentrated way to obtain lycopene, a robust antioxidant that reduces the chance of cardiovascular disease and stroke.

Tomato sauce is a concentrated way to obtain lycopene, a robust antioxidant that reduces the chance of cardiovascular disease and heart stroke. Additionally, some studies also show that lycopene can decrease the threat of osteoporosis. While tomato vegetables generally are saturated in lycopene, cooking food them reduces cell wall space and makes the lycopene more available; adding essential olive oil further raises bioavailability.

Try out this: Make tomato sauce with pumpkin puré electronic, shallots, and stock, add miso paste and puré electronic until clean; simmer tomato sauce with minced onion, garlic clove, Kalamata olives, capers, and anchovies for an easy puttanesca sauce; temperature tomato sauce and cut spinach in a shallow pan, split in eggs, simmer until whites arranged, and provide hot with shaved Parmesan.

6. Tempeh

Like flax, soy contains phytoestrogens that imitate the activities of estrogen and can relieve symptoms of menopause.

Like flax, soy contains phytoestrogens that imitate the activities of estrogen and can relieve symptoms of menopause. Results on the consequences of isoflavones-phytoestrogens in soy-are combined, however, many studies show an advantage to hot adobe flash frequency and/or intensity. In one research, soy reduced hot flashes by 45 percent. Populations with a higher soy consumption likewise have a significant decrease in breasts cancer occurrence, and isoflavones could also have protecting results on cardiovascular and bone health. Soy can be hard to break down, so adhere to tempeh; because it's fermented, tempeh is simpler to process and has an increased content of B nutritional vitamins and increased antioxidant capacity.

Try out this: Stir-fry sliced tempeh with broccolini, thinly sliced onions, shiitake mushrooms, and cashews; simmer crumbled tempeh with onions, peppers, tomato sauce, and seasonings for a vegan sloppy Joe; marinate tempeh cubes in tamari, essential olive oil, and garlic clove natural powder, then bake until crispy for grain-free croutons.

7. Black Beans

Black coffee beans and other legumes contain fiber, which protects against breasts malignancy after menopause.

Black coffee beans and other legumes contain fiber, which protects against breasts malignancy after menopause. They're also abundant with B vitamins, very important to feeling, and magnesium, which protects bone health, enhances sleep, and could relieve panic and depression. Dark coffee beans have higher degrees of antioxidants than other types of coffee beans; they're especially abundant with anthocyanins, which were shown in studies to safeguard against the chance of cardiovascular disease after menopause.

Try out this: Make black coffee beans with shredded special potatoes, chopped kale, and cumin for quick-and-easy breakfast time hash; simmer dark coffee beans with green bell peppers, onions, bay leaves, and oregano, and top with avocado, cilantro, and sour cream; pur é electronic black coffee beans with tahini, essential olive oil, and garlic clove, then mix in finely minced jalapeño peppers for a spicy hummus for snacking.

What Teas Assist With Menopause Symptom Alleviation?

10 teas for menopause relief

Drugs can help balance the hormone changes that occur during perimenopause. Bodily hormones aren't the best option for most women. If you're looking to get more natural and naturopathic remedies, teas may be considered a healthy and less costly option.

While a woman's degrees of estrogen, progesterone, and testosterone drop during menopause, tea can help lessen the symptoms of the changes. Follow bundle instructions (or use approximately 1 teaspoon of tea per 1 cup of warm water) for every serving:

1. Dark cohosh root

Black cohosh main has been found to lessen genital dryness and hot flashes in menopausal women. Research shows that it's most reliable for ladies who experience early menopause. It could be taken in tablet form, or even more popularly, as a tea. It's been used instead of hormone substitute therapy (HRT).

Women who are pregnant shouldn't consume dark cohosh main tea. Those who find themselves being treated for blood circulation pressure or liver organ problems also shouldn't take dark cohosh.

2. Ginseng

Ginseng has shown in reducing the event and intensity of hot flashes and night time sweats in menopausal women. Recent researchTrusted Source has even discovered that it can benefit postmenopausal women reduce their threat of cardiovascular disease. A 2010 research also showed that red ginseng can help menopausal women increase sex arousal and enhance their sex lives.

You are able to drink ginseng tea daily to get its benefits. Taking ginseng as an plant can have many relationships with numerous medications include center, blood circulation pressure, diabetes, and blood-loss medications. Unwanted effects range from jitteriness, head aches, and nervousness.

3. Chasteberry tree

Chasteberry tree has been found to take care of premenstrual symptoms, but taking in the tea can also help simplicity breasts pain (mastodynia) and hot flashes in perimenopausal women.

The herb also increases progesterone, which can help maintain a wholesome balance between estrogen and progesterone throughout the transitions from perimenopause to menopause.

Those using hormones for contraceptive or hormone replacement shouldn't use chasteberry. Aswell, those who've got hormone-sensitive diseases such as breasts malignancy should avoid this tea. That is also wii choice for anybody taking antipsychotic medications or drugs for Parkinson's disease.

4. Red raspberry leaf

Red raspberry leaf tea hasn't been associated with easing common perimenopause symptoms. However, it's a highly effective way to reduce heavy menstrual moves, especially the ones that come at the starting point of perimenopause for most women. This tea is normally considered safe to consider during perimenopause and into menopause.

5. Red clover

Used primarily to take care of hot flashes and evening sweats in women with menopause, red clover in addition has been used to take care of high blood circulation pressure, improve bone strength, and increase immunity. It's generally considered safe. Red clover contains phytoestrogens, a plant-based form of estrogen, which really helps to enhance the hormonal imbalances caused by menopause. This tea is a delicious way to include red clover to your day to day routine.

6. Dong quai

Dong quai tea really helps to balance and regulate estrogen quantity in women entering menopause, reducing or enhancing them depending on your hormonal imbalances.

It has additionally been found to reduce cramps as an indicator of premenstrual symptoms (PMS), and can convenience the pelvic pain in menopause, as well. Avoid this tea if you expect to have surgery. It's been found to hinder blood clotting. People that have fair pores and skin might are more sun delicate after consuming this tea regularly.

A study discovered that the mixture of dong quai and chamomile could reduce hot flashes by up to 96 percentTrusted Source. Learning much more about the advantages of this powerful vegetable.

7. Valerian

Valerian main has health advantages including treating insomnia, anxiety, headaches, and stress. It's been an option for females entering menopause because of its ability to lessen hot flashes.

The herb can also treat joint pain. For ladies experiencing symptoms of osteoporosis, it's rather a great option for enhancing bone strength.

Enjoy a glass of valerian main tea at bedtime to help have a restful night time. Like a tea, there is certainly little risk in taking it. As an natural herb, speak to your doctor first, and steer clear of using it long-term and taking it with alcoholic beverages.

8. Licorice

Licorice tea can help reduce the incident of hot flashes - and exactly how long they last - in women getting into menopause. Additionally, it may have estrogen-like results, and it might be effective in enhancing respiratory health insurance and reducing overall stress.

Licorice can have undesireable effects if blended with certain prescription medications, so seek advice from with a health care provider before consuming.

9. Green tea

A 2009 research revealed that green tea extract can be a highly effective way to strengthen bone metabolism and reduce the threat of bone fractures, especially in women experiencing menopause.

Green tea extract is also filled with antioxidants, some caffeine, and EGCG. EGCG increases metabolism, assisting to battle the putting on weight many menopausal women experience. There is certainly little risk in taking in green tea.

This decaffeinated tea might be considered a good choice if you're concerned about having difficulty sleeping.

10. Ginkgo biloba

Ginkgo biloba has been found to contain phytoestrogens (much like red clover) and can boost estrogen quantity, naturally enhancing hormonal imbalances.

A 2009 research suggested that ginkgo biloba can improve PMS symptoms and the disposition fluctuation that may appear before and during menopause.

Ginkgo biloba tea isn't common, nevertheless, you will get blends like this one that can help. This vitamin can hinder bloodstream clotting, but as a tea for short-term use has little risk.

Are there dangers in taking in these teas?

Check with your doctor before using tea to take care of perimenopause symptoms, since some teas may have undesireable effects on prescription medications. Some teas are natural bloodstream thinners, so consult with a health care provider about your tea utilization, especially before any elective surgery. Periodic use of teas has little risk and may be considered a great option for a mild method of the symptoms of perimenopause.

If you opt to drink tea to fight the symptoms of perimenopause, purchase organic herbal teas, and opt for caffeine-free types since caffeine may get worse menopausal symptoms.

Be cautious with eating the teas hot - particularly if hot flashes are your biggest sign - because they can raise the occurrence of hot flashes and evening sweats. This can be particularly true if you drink them before bed. You are able to brew the tea beforehand and drink it chilly for a cooler substitute.

Other treatments for menopause

If you start to note perimenopausal symptoms, consult with your doctor, who are able to help show you on the best treatment solution.

Hormone alternative therapy (HRT) is cure option for most women. With this program, your physician will recommend you the bodily hormones by means of pills, areas, gels, or lotions. These can help balance your quantity. Based on health and genealogy, however, HRT might not be best for you.

Genital estrogen, which is applied right to the vagina with a cream, tablet, or ring, can help fight genital dryness and discomfort. For females who can't use estrogen therapy, gabapentin (Neurontin) can be a highly effective way to lessen hot flashes.

On the other hand, essential oils could also relieve the symptoms associated with entering menopause when put on differing of your body.

Acknowledgements

The Glory of this book success goes to God Almighty and my beautiful Family, Fans, Readers & well-wishers, Customers, and Friends for their endless support and encouragement.

CPSIA information can be obtained
at www.ICGtesting.com
Printed in the USA
BVHW040945040222
627784BV00027B/1881